ELIZABETH RODDICK

The Other Frontline

The COVID diary of a Community Pharmacist

First edition

Typesetting by Kinga Stabryla

This book was professionally typeset on Reedsy.
Find out more at reedsy.com

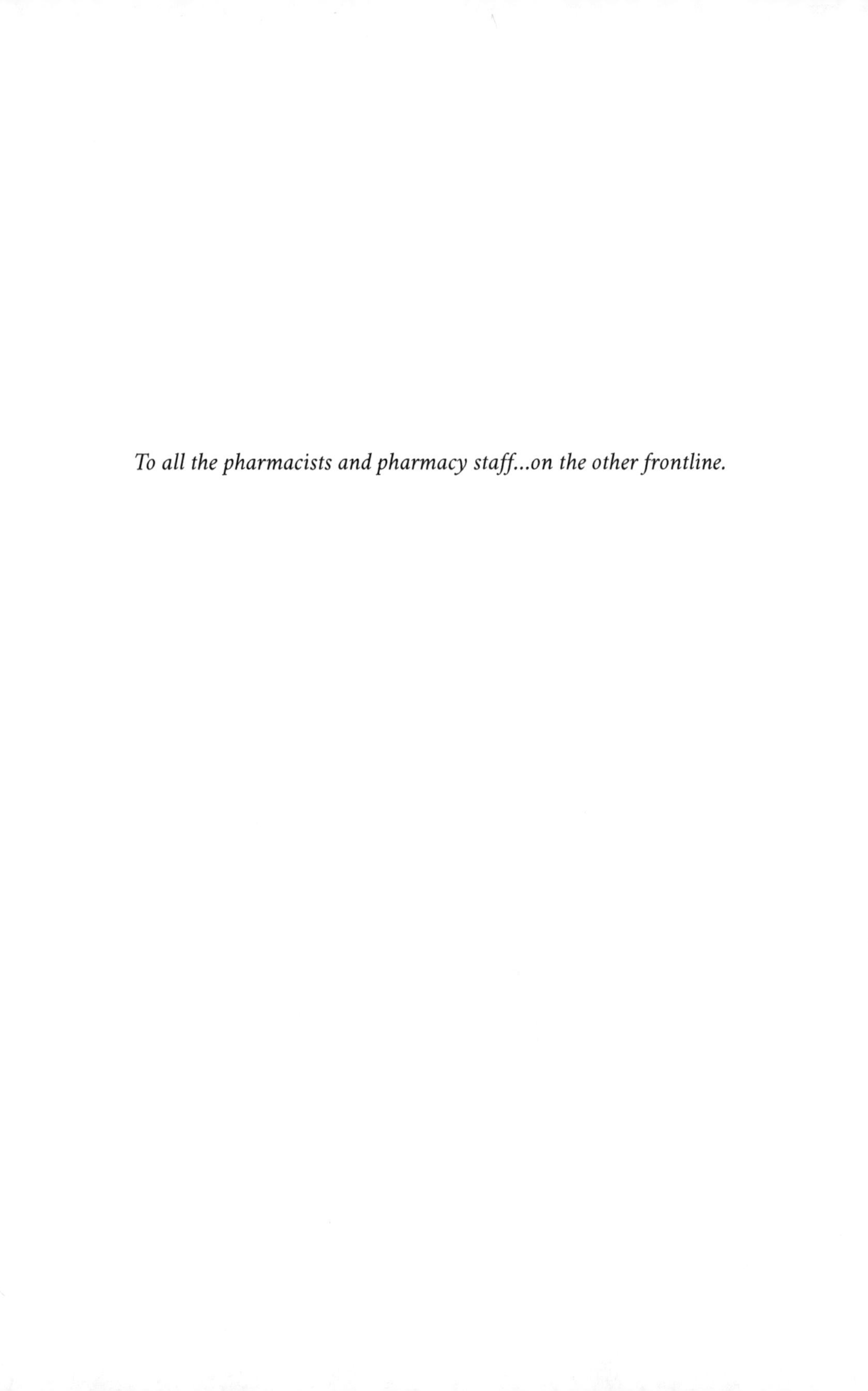

To all the pharmacists and pharmacy staff...on the other frontline.

Contents

1

March

Wednesday 4th March 2020

'Thank you all for attending and contributing to the meeting' the Chair of the Clinical Governance Group at East Renfrewshire Health and Social care Partnership made her closing remarks. It was the 4th March 2020 and little did any of us know what lay ahead.

I arrived back at the pharmacy just after 12 pm to find both phones being used with worried expressions on the faces of my staff.

'Did you hear the news? ' What news?' I answered fearing the worst.

Di was the first to answer. 'India and China are stopping exporting paracetamol.'

'Oh no, that means there's going to be a worldwide shortage. Have you been trying the wholesalers?'

'Yes', this time it was Justyna-'all the wholesalers' paracetamol are marked 'red'. This was our online ordering system and when products showed red that meant they were unavailable.

'Quick get onto our shortline wholesalers and see what they can give us'

'They're rationing Mrs Roddick -you're only allowed 4 dozen and the price has shot up'

'Ok, take them anyway, we'll need to report the prices we are paying - what about the 32's?'

'I can get 4 dozen from Ethigen but again the prices are unbelievable!'

So this was the start of the panic buying. It wasn't toilet rolls in pharmacies, it was paracetamol. The public had obviously heard the news. I'd never seen so many people wanting paracetamol but as well as its being in short supply the Chief Medical Officer had just announced that paracetamol was the best medication to take for Covid-19 symptoms.

Thursday 5th March

An announcement was made that anyone suffering from asthma should make sure they had their inhalers. What happened next was nothing short of a Tsunami.

Anyone who had had an inhaler in the last 10 years was reordering from their GP practice.

Patients who were asking for two of their steroid inhalers were given one with a balance slip explaining that the manufacturers couldn't keep up with demand and, as long as patients had one to keep them going, all was well.

As I looked at the situation in the pharmacy I realised that we as a profession were and are very much at the frontline. We were being swamped with patients both anxious and bewildered trying to get medicines they needed at the start of a pandemic about which we had very little information…

Friday 6th March

I received an e-mail from one of the local GP's. 'Is it possible to get fax numbers and e-mail addresses so that GP's can get in touch if phones are busy?'

I gave her my own details but referred her to the Community Pharmacy Development Team to get all the individual pharmacy information.

Almost simultaneously, the phone rang 'Hello Mrs Roddick, it's Di, my son has a cough and I see from the guidance I'm supposed to self isolate for 14 days.'

'I hope he's alright' I managed to utter but by this time my mind was thinking 'we're getting busier and busier and that's one of my dispenser's off'

'Justyna, can you do some extra hours?'

'Of course, Mrs Roddick' - she was always willing to step up if need be but in the next few days I realised that was going to be far too much of a strain for her.

Monday 9th March

The surgeries were starting to close up and they decided that only pharmacy drivers were allowed to pick up prescriptions. Unfortunately, some surgeries just sent all the prescriptions where it was marked 'collect by the patient' to one or two pharmacies and they quickly became overwhelmed.

'Can we close at lunchtime and a bit earlier at night so we can catch up?' was the cry from many pharmacies in order to cope with the massive increase in workload.

The Health Board Implementation Group started to put out notices to overwhelmed pharmacies. 'Yes you can shorten your model hours 9-5.30/6 and you can take a lunchtime break'.

I decided that we would stay open but at what cost? As I looked at the situation in the pharmacy I realised that we as a profession were very exposed so I wrote to the Herald who amazingly enough published my letter about the need for masks and general recognition of the community pharmacists and the headline by the editor was :

'Pharmacists are on the frontline in the coronavirus fight and must be protected.'

Wednesday 11th March

Medicine shortages were taking a lot of time up. Each drug had to be sourced often not from our usual wholesalers but sometimes from a colleague.

A nearby colleague dealt with another Phoenix wholesaler-'Can you check if you can get Nozinan'?

This is a palliative care drug which all network pharmacies (of which New Life is one) need to have in stock.

'Yes' said Ian and we discussed what stock we would swap when my driver arrived over at his pharmacy.

Getting stock was proving difficult plus our wholesalers were suggesting cutting down on deliveries as they had seen a drop in available drivers.

Friday 13th March

'Have you got that cement to put my cap back in?' This was a chap who insisted in showing me the massive gap at the front of his teeth showing two stumps .'I've phoned the manufacturers and they say they are overwhelmed - it's going to be some time before they can produce the product. I'll put your name on a list if you like?' I answered.

He thanked me, grimaced and left the pharmacy quite troubled.

Dentists were locking their doors so we were getting more and more queries about general mouth and teeth problems.

Sunday 15th March

Sunday should be a day off but I decided to go into the pharmacy and try and clear up. There were boxes of extra stockpiled up since, anytime a medicine that was in the short category was available, we ordered as many as we were allowed. I felt very tired but also a sense of satisfaction since clearing up was almost therapeutic-yes we would have a good start next week or so I thought.

Tuesday 17th March

Things were getting busier and busier and I was wondering how we were going to get through all the prescriptions when I received another call this time it was Tracey.

'Mrs Roddick my son has a cough and I've been told to take him out of school and self-isolate for 14 days.'

'Do you think he has the virus? 'No' said Tracey but the school says we can't take any chances.' This would have been a good time to have testing in place for frontline workers.

I wished her and her son well and then fixed my mind on how we were going to keep the pharmacy open. 'Two dispensers down' I thought and I looked at Justyna who was nervous anyway about the virus and was beginning to show signs of panic.

I reached for the phone 'Eileen - is there any chance of you coming into the pharmacy?'

Eileen, a locum pharmacist had been covering my meetings, days off and holidays for the past while and, after explaining my predicament, there was no hesitation.

'Yes, of course, I'll be there in 20 minutes.'

Talk about a knight in shining armour. Eileen got straight onto the pile of dispensed items waiting to be checked and by this time we had moved basket after basket containing the prescriptions along with labelled medicines into the consulting room. 'When will I be using this room again for consultations?' I thought

Adam, my pharmacy student and Neil my assistant also managed to do some well-needed shifts.

What was so gratifying was the number of offers of help from patients. 'Can I come in and help in the back or do you need prescriptions delivered?

I explained that staff in the pharmacy had all been rigorously trained before being allowed to dispense and similarly, drivers all had to have checks and follow particular procedures.

'Thank you for all your offers of help though.' I kept saying to each patient.

Thursday 19th March

'Alan (our driver) can you go into that hardware shop up the road and get as many of these plastic baskets as you can?' The plastic baskets are so that each individual prescription can be dispensed ready for checking by the pharmacist. This has always been an important safety feature and, as we were rapidly running out of them it was a priority to purchase some more.

Alan arrived back in half an hour and we started using them right away for the massive bundle of prescriptions.

'Do you have any paracetamol?' 'Yes' I replied but I need to pack it down from 100 pack, Can you give me your details please?' Every five minutes there was another request for the medicine. There had been another announcement that paracetamol was the drug of choice for Covid symptoms and in fact, ibuprofen might worsen the situation. (This was subsequently disproved). 'Justyna, can you check our stock and start phoning round to get some more?' I didn't want to run out of this important medicine.

Panic buying was starting for gloves, hand sanitisers, masks and thermometers. This pandemic was changing peoples' lives. They were becoming scared and looking for reassurance.

Saturday 21st March

How was I going to keep the pharmacy staff safe? I telephoned a colleague who had erected a partial perspex screen. By this time we had been told to practise social distancing. My husband brought a folding table into the pharmacy and erected it in front of the counter to increase the distance. We also fixed a tape on the floor two meters back from the counter with 'x's at 2-meter distances.

'Good morning here are your deliveries' Paul from AAH had always been very polite and cheery as he brought the orders into the dispensary. I began to realise that wholesale drivers generally could possibly be carrying the virus in with them so I started the rule that they would leave the boxes at the front and only controlled drugs would be handed to pharmacists for checking. I also suggested that staff wear gloves when handling the 'totes'-the boxes that wholesalers use for transporting the drugs and also when handling cardboard in case of transmission from surfaces. We also had our first of many meetings that Wednesday about safety in the pharmacy getting risk assessments drawn up.

Wednesday 25th March

'I'm not happy when patients come right up and lean over the table' said Justyna. 'Yes', I replied, 'I'm exploring getting a perspex screen built.'

'Bryan (our local joiner) can you meet my husband at the pharmacy to discuss erecting a screen to keep patients and staff safe?'

Bryan arrived the next day and discussed (keeping the 2-meter distance) with my husband how he envisaged the screen would look.

'You're going to have to work when the pharmacy's closed' I said.

'Yes' said Brian' but maybe I could build some of it in my workshop.'

We agreed that he would come in two days later after work.

It meant I was at work to almost 9 pm two nights in a row but I knew that many of my colleagues were doing the same.

Friday 27th March

There was a problem with the setup.

'But how were we going to get prescriptions in and out plus the card machine with the large screen between us and our patients?

'You see that old tea trolley we got as a wedding present?' my husband said to me that night.

'I looked over at the trolley which had several plants dangling from its surface.'

'It will certainly need a clean and how do we get it back and forth?'

'Here you are' Douglas had found a piece of rope with hooks-'we'll hook it up and you can push it forward and pull it back-I think it will work well'

Little did I know that the trolley was going to catch the imagination of the online community and in fact the BBC.

Monday 30th March

It became apparent early on that community pharmacists were dealing with many more queries than normal. ' I have bloodshot eyes', 'I have an ulcer in my mouth', 'could you look at my rash?' The queries were endless because we as a profession were still easily accessible.

The chap with the gap at the front of his mouth came back.

'Do you think super glue would work for my caps?' 'Oh no, please don't use that, it's full of chemicals. Look the minute I get the dental cement I'll phone you - promise.'

It seemed to me that my staff and I were taking on extra duties.

'Can you stand in the window for a minute 'till this patient comes round to get his medication?' I felt like a traffic warden directing patients so that everyone kept two meters apart. It was an ongoing effort to try and keep patients and staff safe.

Keeping the dozens of weekly trays for patients going was really difficult but thankfully the East Renfrewshire Health and Social Care Partnership loaned me a dispenser for a day to try and catch up.

2

April

Wednesday April 1st

The next query was a man who'd fallen outside. His glasses had penetrated his forehead and he was losing quite a lot of blood. Social distancing was not going to work with this emergency. I donned some surgical gloves and led the man into the consulting room where I rinsed out his wound with sterile saline and applied a thick pad to the wound.'I want you to press really hard on the pad -take a seat out in the front shop and I'll phone your surgery.'

I explained the situation to the receptionist who then told me that the best place for the patient to go was the Queen Elizabeth Minor Injuries Department.

'Can I phone you a taxi?' I shouted through the perspex, 'and if you need cash you can hand it back after you're recovered.'

'Thanks so much ' he said as he headed out the door to the taxi.

Friday April 3rd

A box of chocolates was placed on the trolley. 'Just to let you know' said the gentleman 'that I needed seven stitches in my forehead. It will probably mean my film appearances will be curtailed ' he said with a wink.

'Glad to see you are well' I replied and I know the staff all like chocolates, 'thank you.'

'No thank you' he said as he walked out.

The next problem to appear was a mother with her young son. 'I was told by the receptionist that you could maybe look at his face?'

At this point, I found a new use for the trolley. 'Right Seon, I want you to hold onto the trolley and push it forward until I say stop.' That way I was able to look at his face but still maintain some distance between us.

Yes, it was impetigo. After that, I was able to go through a few questions with the mother including hygiene requirements then issue a prescription for fusidic acid cream.

'Will you bring Seon in after five days to let me see how things are?'

'Sure, thank you' said the mother and left.

Saturday April 4th

'Mrs Roddick-there's a phone call from a man wondering if you could do a tetanus jag?'

'Hello? Can you not get that done at minor injuries?', 'No' said the man 'the Victoria is shut and I'm not going to the Queen Elizabeth's.'

As I had all the Patient Group Direction qualifications and being an independent prescriber it was certainly legal for me to do the injection.

'You will have to wear a mask' I said and then I looked at my own PPE -a mask and apron and wondered if it was wise for me to do this. I did surmise though that all through the pandemic it had not always been possible to keep social distancing with patients.

The gentleman thanked me profusely after getting the vaccine.

' Not at all' I said but thought ' It seems that once again pharmacy was being asked to do even more'.

Wednesday 8th April

'The doctor's surgery asked me to bring in my little girl for you to look at her rash.' said the young woman in front of me.

I found out the girl's name was Krissie. 'Mum, would it be alright if Krissie comes along to the end of the chairs and you stand back so that it's only the child I'm close to?' 'Sure' said the mother and thankfully Krissie was at an age that she did what she was told and complied. I looked at the mother. 'Where is the rash?'

The mother didn't have to answer since Krissie had already lifted up her jumper above her head. 'It's on my tummy' she said defiantly.

I had a good look then asked the usual questions about how long Krissie had had it, had she had it before, was it anywhere else on the body and was she well in herself - no temperature or stiff neck?'

As all of these answers pointed to an allergy we then discussed a change of soap powder or had she been playing outside maybe lying on grass?

With the questions answered in a satisfactory way, I prescribed some antihistamine on a Pharmacy First prescription and asked the mother to bring Krissie in after a few days and let me see how she is. With the usual caveat of 'if things change and you're worried, seek medical help' Krissie and her mother left.

Saturday 11th April

'I've run out of my blood pressure tablets and the doctors are shut.' the lady in front of me explained. 'Do you normally get your prescription here?' I asked. 'No' said the lady 'but my regular pharmacy has a half-day on a Saturday.' 'Do you have an empty packet with you?

'No' said the lady 'I don't know the name but it was a yellow box.'

I realised I would have to get the actual name of the medication before issuing an emergency supply.

'If you give me permission to look at your medical notes then that will tell me what medicine you are on.'

Thankfully, pharmacists are now able to access, with the patient's permission, their Emergency Care Summary.

Yes, it was Amlodipine 5mg so I prescribed the medicine using the Unscheduled Care service and produced a prescription. This would then be sent to the patient's doctor to let him or her know that the patient had received the medicine.

Tuesday 14th April

The mobile phone was carefully placed on the trolley as I pulled the object towards me. Here was a picture of someone's mouth. It showed a large ulcer on the inside of the person's lip. 'It's my husband's. He's gone to work and asked me to call in,'

'Is there any way I could speak to him?'

Armed with his phone number I headed into the consulting room to get some key questions answered.

'Yes, I think I burnt my mouth a couple of days ago. No, I only have a drink at weekends.'

So with a promise from the young man to seek dental help if it didn't clear up I gave his wife some steroid tablets to dissolve on the ulcer. (I heard later that that had been very successful).

Monday 20th April

The first telephone call was from a dentist. 'Can you dispense a prescription for one of my patients? It's for Amoxycillin?' 'Of course, give me all the details and we'll get it ready right away.'

The dentist was remarking that his hands were tied during the lockdown. He was working from home and the only thing he could offer patients was a prescription.

Of course, anything more serious could be dealt with in the hubs that are being set up.

I commiserated with him and wished him well.

Yes, lots of services were being put on hold.

The next woman wanted the morning after pill so I was able to take her once again into the private area with the social distancing rule in place. One of the important services we can do as well as prescribing the tablet, if appropriate, is to counsel on ongoing contraception and protection against sexually transmitted diseases.

Wednesday 29th April

'Could you look at this rash on my body?' said the young man at the pharmacy entrance.

I signalled to the gentleman outside to wait while I came round to examine his torso. There was the telltale sign of a shingles rash so I asked him how it felt. 'When my shirt touches it's very sore.' 'Ok. I'm going to prescribe a tablet which I want you to take five times a day. I'll write out the times because it's really important to take it this way and to complete the course. That will hopefully mean that there won't be any residual nerve pain afterwards.'

He thanked me and left.

The next lady mouthed to me that she thought she had a urine infection and that the surgery suggested she came into the pharmacy.

I took her into the semi-private area and asked her several questions to ascertain that it was an uncomplicated urinary tract infection and that I could therefore safely prescribe for her. All was well and the lady left clutching her three days course of trimethoprim.

<h1 style="text-align:center">3</h1>

<h1 style="text-align:center">May</h1>

Monday 4th May

The Scottish Government had asked community pharmacists to open on the May holidays as well as GP's so this was the first of the May holidays.

I thought that, since we would be quiet, I would only ask my most inexperienced member of staff to work letting the others have a well-earned rest.

I couldn't have been more wrong in terms of how busy it would be. I had told the Health Board personnel I would open from 11 am to 4 pm.

Knowing it was better to prepare early I was ready at 10 am with both computers on and stock on shelves and in drawers waiting to see what the day would bring.

At exactly 11 am the phone started ringing. This was a receptionist phoning in prescriptions from a surgery. What was amazing was that the phone didn't stop ringing and people were coming into the pharmacies with a multitude of questions.

Some of the prescriptions had to be delivered. I telephoned home 'Douglas, with Alan being off can you so some deliveries?'

As usual, he obliged.

Although we were supposed to close at 4 pm it was 6 pm when I let my staff member go. What a day it had been and taught me a lesson that during the pandemic, holiday Monday opening required a full staff complement.

Tuesday 5th May

I realised I was feeling exhausted then it dawned on me that I had been working for 63 days including Sundays without a break. I phoned my locum- could she work tomorrow, the 6th, to allow me to have a day off? 'Of course' said Eileen and so I battled on through the day knowing that I would be able to rest on Wednesday. That was a lifesaver.

Thursday 7th May

'I've got a really sore foot' said the middle-aged woman from behind the screen. I came out to the front so that I could observe the problem.'Yes, I'm afraid you have an infection. Ok, I'll prescribe some antibiotics for you and inform your surgery. I need to take all your details and you must come back in 5 days to let me see how the infection is clearing.'

When she did come back in I decided she needed a further five days treatment and thankfully that did the trick.

That was another patient that didn't need to be seen by a doctor. My independent prescribing course was starting to come into its own.

And the deliveries were increasing every day. The East Renfrewshire Hub had set up a prescription delivery service plus many patients had come in to ask if they could deliver as well. We were very grateful for the offers of assistance but we just kept going with the resources we had. Alan's hours almost doubled on a daily basis with patients shielding but, along with my back up husband's help, they seemed to cope. A grateful thanks to both of them.

Friday 8th May

'We just can't seem to get the HRT patch for this lady' said Eileen when she was in looking through the prescriptions in the 'balance basket'. These prescriptions contained all the drugs that were on a short supply. Pharmacists spend a lot of time trying to source alternative stock and liaising with GP surgeries with alternative suggestions.

'We decided to e-mail the surgery with the suggestion of an alternative patch plus a capsule for the progesterone part of the original prescription.' I said to the patient in front of me.

The lady looked a little panicked at that point.

'Don't worry we will get you an alternative -it just might take a couple of days.'

'But I've run out' said the lady with a perplexed expression.. 'Ok I'll personally phone the practice with my suggestion and tell them it needs to be sorted today if possible.'

'If you come back at around six o'clock-we close at six-thirty I hope to have your medication ready.'

'Thanks' said the lady and yes, the surgery came up trumps and gave me the new script over the phone just before they closed.

Monday 11th May

Alan, the driver arrived in with a bottle of wine and a box of chocolates. 'This is from Mrs Smith-you seemingly helped her get the right make of medicine for her little girl.'

I'm always amazed by the generosity of patients when I think we are just doing our job.

'There are another four deliveries Alan-can you manage that?'

'Yes of course but can I have a chocolate to keep my strength up?'

'Yes', I said 'choose the one you want.'

'Can you deliver this medicine?' said the receptionist from one of the local surgeries. I looked at my watch - it was now 5.30 in the afternoon and I realised it would have to be myself doing the delivery 'Yes of course' I said with a slight sinking feeling with it turning out to be a very long day.

I was glad I had delivered since, even with the two-meter distance, after I had deposited the medicine on the front doorstep, the elderly lady looked far from well when she gave me a wave from the door.

Wednesday 13th May

'We're doing a feature on 'high tech/low tech' regarding social distancing and keeping people safe' said Gillian Sharp on the phone. 'We'd like to film your trolley and maybe do an interview with you and some patients.'

I guessed early on that I was the 'low tech' part of the piece since smart apple watches and the like were labelled 'high tech'

We agreed that the filming would take place the following Friday early morning so as not to disrupt the work of the pharmacy.

Friday 15th May

In the BBC personnel came with a camera, a microphone on an extended pole for social distancing and a list of 'shots' that would need to be taken.

The sound engineer was down kneeling on the floor at one point 'Can you roll the trolley back and forward?' 'Yes', I said thinking he had gone a little mad but then he explained 'We're going to do a piece for Radio Scotland as well.'

It was an interesting experience making BBC Scotland's 'Mornings' radio show and the lunchtime BBC Scotland's national news.

What wasn't so good was the number of young women telling me that their grandmother had one of these trolleys!

I spent the next few days reflecting on this amazing Covid 19 experience. One thing I did realise was that it was only because of the hard work of my staff and my locum that helped me play a part in this pandemic.

Also, I can honestly say that it's been a privilege to serve my patients in the community over this troubled time and thanks to them for their support.

WHAT WILL THE NEXT 90 DAYS BRING?

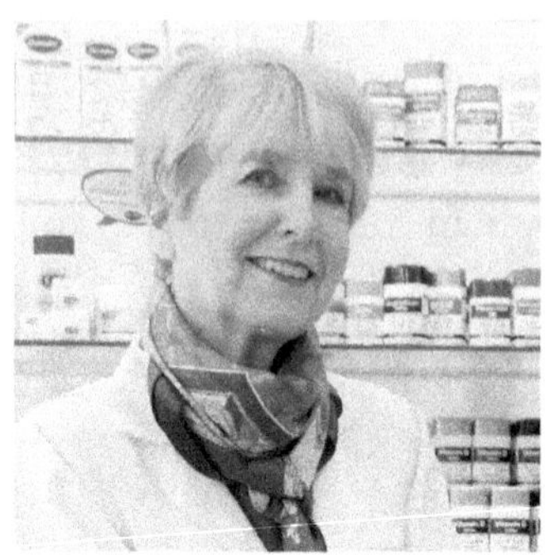

About the Author

An NHS Award-winning pharmacist, Elizabeth Roddick, is the writer of the #1 Amazon bestseller 'Call The Pharmacist'.

The book is a very personal account of her life in and out of her community 'New Life Pharmacy' that she owns and manages. Starting with her father's struggle as a chemist in 1938, she details the rich, humorous and sometimes poignant stories of the interaction with her patients and customers. The development of pharmacy services over the 30 year period is illustrated on top of demonstrating her holistic approach to health within her pharmacy and in the public speaking arena.

She is a weekly contributor to RNIB Connect Radio, where she broadcasts her 'Call the Pharmacist' slot. She can also be heard on BBC Radio Scotland's Call Kaye programme answering questions on health topics. Occasionally, Elizabeth can be heard speaking about the holistic side of health, as well as GP educational topics at venues such as the London Expo Centre, the Edinburgh Fringe, the Edinburgh Science Festival and community events.

She is a Fellow of the Royal Pharmaceutical Society (RPS) having been the Chair of the Scottish Executive of the RPS and has held various positions in pharmacyprofessionalbodiesthroughouthercareer.

Youcanconnectwithmeon:
http://elizabethroddick.com
https://www.facebook.com/CallThePharmacistUK

Also by Elizabeth Roddick

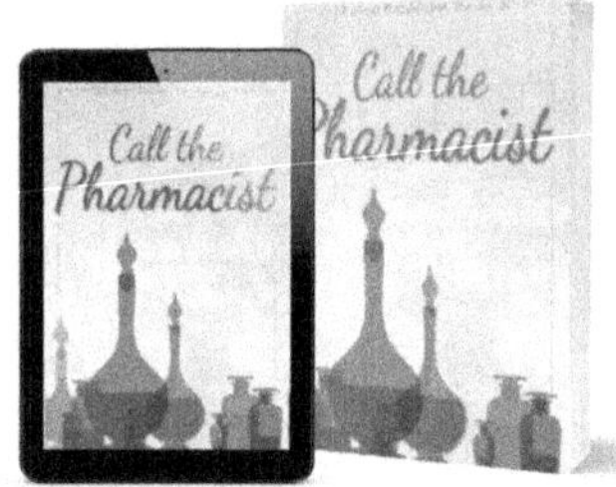

Call the Pharmacist

Set in Glasgow, Elizabeth Roddick, an NHS award-winning pharmacist, gives a very personal account of her life in and out of her community pharmacy. Starting with her father's struggle as a chemist in 1938, she details the rich, humorous and sometimes poignant stories of the interaction with her patients and customers. The development of pharmacy services over the 30 year period is illustrated as well as demonstrating her holistic approach to health within her pharmacy and in the public speaking arena.